I0455807

Copyright © 2017

Ordering Information:

Quantity sales. Special discounts are available on quantity purchases
by corporations, associations, and others. Orders by U.S. trade
bookstores and wholesalers.

Printed in the United States of America

First Printing, 2017

ISBN-13: 978-1547294732

ISBN-10: 1547294736

# Disclaimer (My Lawyer Made Me Write This):

*"I am not a doctor by any means. We therefore advise you to consult a doctor before attempting using Spinner Fidgets for therapeutic benefits!"*

# Learning to Love Your Body

"Your body is precious. It is our vehicle for awakening. Treat it with care." ~Buddha

Let's start off this journey together. I am here for you. I originally did not start out by writing this book. This is a collection of my blog posts I have been writing for the last year. But I have had so much positive feedback from my wonderful followers that I wanted to turn it into a book.

The purpose of this book is to educate you on the great many benefits of using a spinner fidget – for you and your child. It has completed changed my daughter's life. You see, Elli was diagnosed with severe anxiety, since the age of 6, and had trouble coping in school. Her grades fell, had trouble maintaining friendships, and become detached. Children can be harsh towards one another and she was made fun of a lot.

We visited all the best doctors around and even tried all the current medication out there. We've tried everything including some essential oils and none of it has worked. After not achieving much success, I turned towards holistic medicine as a long shot. Long story short, I heard about these fidget spinners, on Facebook of all places! People were using to cure anxiety. I was skeptical at first how a little toy could help anyone get better until I personally tried it. However, over time, it calmed down my restless sleep and anxiety. I can't tell you how happy I was to have a non-medication alternative to give to my daughter. The toy cured her anxiety within about one week of trying it. Let me just tell you this… It has made the different between night and day. I also struggled with depression and anxiety for many years and decided to use the spinner for my own benefit. I continue to use it today. I can't describe how much better I feel after a long stressful day at work.

It's now become a habit, where it's the one thing that I look forward to at night to relax before going to bed. I wrap up in a blanket and listen to soft music and I feel so "Special"! I spin the dam spinner. I sip a nice glass of wine. It's nice to pamper oneself after a long day of doing and going. It gives you the calming feeling and I can't help but feel so relaxed. It's like reading a good book, and dying to get to the next chapter, as it's that good and you've just got to know more... I absolutely love it and wish that I could say more, but it's now my time to go get this blanket on and get pampered!!!"

## The Origins of a Spinner Fidgets

Attention Deficit Hyperactivity Disorder (ADHD) is the most common behavioral disorder diagnosed in children. Common signs include restlessness, continual talking and inability to concentrate and pay attention. About 18% of school-aged children have been diagnosed with ADHD, with 1 in 3 having received treatment with medication and behavioral therapy. A lot of these students end up falling behind their peers academically.

# New Insight into Hyperactivity

In my research, I found a new study published in The Journal of Abnormal Child Psychology which suggests that hyperactivity may actually help students overcome their attention problems. Common hyperactive behaviors like running, jumping, rolling on the floor and continual talking are typically viewed as a disruptive problem that should be treated in addition to the attention problems. Researchers found that when students with ADHD were asked to perform a task that involved working memory and organization, those who were allowed to move or fidget did significantly better than those who were asked to keep still. Conversely, children without ADHD did better when sitting still, but worse when moving around.

Many feel these findings suggest that students with ADHD actually *need* their gross motor movements to help them complete challenging intellectual tasks. Rather than being part of the problem, it's likely that hyperactive behaviors help these students stay focused and attend to the task at hand. Researchers describe "excess motor activity as a compensatory mechanism that facilitates neurocognitive functioning in children with ADHD." This means that hyperactivity may be a feature to encourage rather than a bug to fix.

# Effective Teaching

I believe the reason why fidget spinners are not allowed in many classrooms is because traditional classroom management programs try to get rid of or eliminate disruptive behavior, these findings require some new thinking about how to effectively teach students with ADHD. It's a major challenge to maintain a learning environment that respects the needs of traditional learners who thrive in quiet, orderly spaces while allowing students with ADHD the freedom to move. Student safety is also important, so it's crucial for teachers to create a classroom with designated times and spaces for movement. Some strategies for teachers to employ in the classroom include:

Allowing students to keep a fidget toy in their desks is a small start. Students can take the toy out when they feel like interrupting or jumping up. This can be a ball to squeeze or another toy with interesting tactile properties to keep them physically engaged so they can pay attention. Designating a corner of the classroom as an "Activity Zone" or a "Jumping Corner" creates a place where students can retreat when they feel the need to move around. This area is ideally placed in the back of the room where other students will not be distracted, but will allow clear sight lines to the teacher so the student can continue to follow the lesson.

A yoga ball chair or therapy bands tied to chair legs can help students with ADHD bounce and move without leaving their seats. This is especially effective during tests or writing sessions that require quiet thinking and movement at the same time.

As more research indicates that hyperactive behavior helps students with ADHD overcome concentration struggles to master complex material, it's more important than ever for teachers to find creative ways that support these students within their comfort zones. Allowing students to fidget in a controlled, respectful way can improve academic performance and create a classroom environment that is more comfortable for all learners.

These fidget spinners help kids focus and also helps with stress. You will find that many kids think they are really fun. The palm-sized device, which can be spun with a flick of a finger, may be advertised as a way to improve concentration and reduce anxiety. But spinners have also become the hot toy among elementary- and middle-school students. Not all teachers agree on the device's benefits, and schools in some districts are trying to keep the spinners out of the classroom.

Administrators will confiscate them because they think they are highly distracting. They think it looks like a toy but little do they know it is a device intended to help children focus.

The fidget spinner is a device that offer a sensory outlet for children with ADD, ADHD and Autism Spectrum Disorder. There's no research on the actual fidget spinners yet and research on fidgets for kids on their desk at school is actually very poor. Studies show physical activity helps children with ADHD concentrate, but most research focuses on the use of large muscle groups, not fine motor skills. But unfortunately, there just isn't a whole heck of a lot of data to support that they're effective. Fidgets also may be distracting to other students in the classroom, particularly among other children with ADHD, she said. Though more research is needed to determine the effectiveness of fidgets some believe they help. I definitely do believe it.

I can't explain why it works, but it does. Just trust me

Mental health experts have been using similar toys for years. In fact, the Slinky is one of the earliest fidget toys. It's not a massive surprise – they've become somewhat of a craze recently, and it seems like all kids are spinning them around and occasionally throwing them their classmates. But what schools that have issues the bans are missing is how much of a help fidget spinners and cubes can be for students with anxiety, ADHD, and other mental health issues. Fidget spinners and fidget cubes have been popping up in anxiety groups on Facebook and touted as remedies for overwhelming worries for a while now, but it's only fairly recently that parents have discovered their benefits for kids.

The clicking, spinning, and twirling children and adults can do with fidget spinners and cubes help to keep hands busy and provide a distraction or sensory stimulation for those with specific mental health issues.

Yes, they can distract from lessons – but they'll also distract from anxiety or trauma symptoms, and can soothe children with sensory issues. Without being able to use these products, these children will likely be unable to focus on lessons: but because of their mental health struggles, not the subtle clicking away of a pocket-size cube.

The idea of fidget spinner therapy is far from new. It is from a branch of study, called deep-touch therapy and it goes back to a basic human behavior known to calm us — being held. Clinical studies suggest that when certain pressure points on the body are stimulated by touch, the brain releases a chemical called serotonin. This neurotransmitter is responsible for regulating various brain functions, including sleep and mood.

The key to this stimulation is the rare weight (heaviness) of the spinner, which is able to create a deep pressure. Aside from swaddles, this kind of pressure is present in hugs and when we stroke animals or our loved ones. On the opposite side of the spectrum, light touch pressure is a more superficial stimulation of the skin, such as tickling, very light touch, or moving hairs on the skin and provide no therapeutic benefits at all. Occupational therapists have observed that a very light touch alerts the nervous system, but deep pressure is relaxing and calming. This is why the fidget spinners work.

## A MULTI-USE THERAPY

Back in the day, I found out that deep touch pressure stimulation was used to help children with ADHD. These kids often experience sensory overload, meaning they have difficulty filtering out background sensory information. This can cause restlessness, anxiety, and trouble participating in seated activities and ongoing tasks. Of course, sleeping can be difficult in this state as well. Study after study has shown fidget spinners can help children with ASD fall asleep. The kids benefit not only from the release of serotonin the blankets bring, but also from the decrease in heart rate and blood pressure that result from the calming effect. This allows for more control, and in turn, a better chance of rest.

Fidget spinners and deep-touch pressure benefits those without a specific sensory disorder as well. After I recommended them to family members and friends, they all came back to me with positive stories and results. Loved ones who were complaining of sleep dysfunction, stress, and pain had better overall better sleep quality and reported lower anxiety. Please note, I am not a doctor, but since the therapy is safe, patients with a multitude of conditions have given spinners a try and magically cured within a week too. I've researched study after study and found 95% of its participates with post-traumatic stress disorder, obsessive-compulsive disorder, attention deficit hyperactivity disorder, and all types of anxiety had positive results as well.

Spinners can provide a feeling of calm and comfort that has escaped some for a long time The weight of the blanket acts as deep touch therapy.

# Anxiety

Anxiety Disorder is a term used to describe a broad range of different anxiety-producing issues. While we all might experience a bout of anxiety from time to time, it becomes a disorder when the fear is prolonged over months, or even years, consistently or episodically. It can be advantageous having a spinner fidget around to use you begin to feel the onset of a panic attack, irritability, or a lack of concentration.

There are many types of brand names on the market today. I'm not here to endorse a specific one. Please do your research before purchasing a blanket.

## 10 Therapeutic Benefits

Many seniors, adults, teenagers and children face psychiatric issues that cause severe anxiety. Patients with autism and other psychiatric disorders also face extreme anxiousness and the inability to induce calmness within themselves without the use of sedatives or drugs.

The root causes of such behavioral issues are anxiety and insomnia, which is usually treated with pharmacological (drugs) and psychological (therapy) methods. However, now with a breakthrough in the study of sleep medicine and psychiatric disorders, we know that the trick to soothing consternation and inducing sleep is much simpler than we thought.

The drug-free therapeutic fidget spinners have become the at-home treatment for insomnia, anxiety, autism spectrum disorders (ASD), attention-deficit hyperactive disorders (ADHD), Restless Leg Syndrome (RLS), Asperger's and sensory disorders. Spinners use deep pressure touch simulation (DPTS) to relax the body and make the patient feel safe, guarded and secure, which calms their unease and helps their body go to sleep. The sensory compression methodology facilitates a positive change with the comfort the blanket brings to its user. The weight of the spinner stimulates the receptors on your body which then activates the neurotransmitters in your brain to bring a sense of happiness to the person. This spinner has shown to be very effective in calming hyperactive children during bedtime, anxious patients in therapy and even adults undergoing chemotherapy. It has also proven to be efficacious in calming people down during anxiety inducing situations.

From my research, some of the therapeutic benefits of the spinners are given below.

## 1. Promotes Sleep

Insomnia is a sleep disorder that causes sleeplessness. The lack of sleep leads to the over exhaustion of the body and hampers the psychological well-being of the person. When a person is not able to function well, both physically and mentally, their social wellbeing is affected and they begin to lose productivity in their lives. This leads to depression and other behavioral problems.

An easy solution to this problem is the fidget spinner. The pressure reaches deep within the body of the user to provide a comfortable environment for a person to fall asleep in. The sense of being swaddled and the physical connection that the user feels with the blanket makes them feel warm and safe. This helps their mind be at ease and they can be able to relax their body. The state of tranquility will help clear their mind and ensure a good night's sleep.

## 2. Imitates a Warm Hug

Research shows that hugs can actually make a person feel at ease. Hugging a person releases the hormone Oxytocin into the blood stream. This chemical reduces your blood pressure, calms your heart rate and provides and overall feeling of relaxation. Although the spinner does not provide a human connection, your body may perceive the warmth and security the imitation that a hug provides. Both the hug and the spinner use a gentle yet firm pressure that goes deep within the person's body tissues. This gives the user a sense of repose and allows your body to relax.

## 3. Sense of Security

As mentioned above, the feel of the spinner will ensure the feeling of calmness in the user. The 'blanket therapy' stimulates the receptors present throughout our body, which lessens a person's discomfort. Once the user feels more comfortable in the blanket, they begin to feel secure as their body begins to relax. The body can only relax when your mind is soothed and your heart rate is calmed. This change in the body will ensure that both your body and mind believes that you are secure and safe.

## 4. Increases the Production of Serotonin

Serotonin is a chemical messenger, also known as a neurotransmitter that your brain and intestines produce for the smooth functioning of your nervous system, which includes the brain and the nerves. This hormone is secreted to promote happiness and the mood of the people. Known as the 'happy hormone', this chemical does not only affect a person's mood but it affects their behavior. The lack of serotonin in the body leads to depression, insomnia and anxiety. That is why the sensory stimulating spinners increase the production of serotonin in the body. The hormone relaxes your body and makes you feel calmer. That sense of calmness leads to pacifying one's anxiety, which results to inducing sleep in the user.

## 5. Increase in the Production of Melatonin

Melatonin, also known as the 'sleep hormone' is a chemical that affects a person's sleep. The hormone is produced with the production of serotonin, as well as the pineal gland in the brain. This chemical is known to ease insomnia and induce sleep, which is possible through the therapeutic benefits of the weighted blankets that provide a gentle yet firm pressure on your body by stimulating your receptors.

## 6. Calms Patients with Autism Spectrum Disorder

Autism spectrum disorder includes Asperger's, Autism, Rhett Syndrome and other unspecified Pervasive Development Disorders. Such disorders include behavioral problems that do not necessarily bode well with the norms of society. The patients suffering from such disorders feel aggression and irritation due to the inability to express or convey their thoughts clearly. Such slow cognitive development makes the patient unable to process information quickly and the change in their surroundings. Patients with such disorders are not able to communicate properly, so they use erratic speech, repetitive actions and turbulent behaviors. During a frustrated outburst, the patient's heart rate increases, their breath becomes shallow and their blood pressure rises – which further increases their irritability.

When the patient is going through such tempestuous emotions and tantrums, it is best to use the spinner around them or have them lay down with the blanket covering them. This will make them feel more relaxed and comfortable. Once they are no longer acting in a hysterical manner, they will be able to think with a clearer mind and a calmer body. Although communicating with their caretakers might still be difficult, there will at least be an opportunity for the patient to gather more patience and attempt to convey their thoughts in a more serene manner.

## 7. Helps Overcome the Oversensitivity to Touch

Some psychiatric disorders make people oversensitive to touch. Patients with Autism Spectrum Disorders usually face such discomfort with the touch of other people but this can be overcome by introducing the weight of the blanket regularly to the affected patient. The pressure of the spinner provides a similar feeling of human touch at a larger scale without actual connection – which can be a stepping stone in helping patients overcome their fear of touch.

During the 1990s, a squeeze machine was used to help patients overcome their oversensitivity to touch. Today, with the inception of the 'therapy blankets', patients can use the more accessible and less controversial mechanism to help people become more at ease with touch.

## 8. Pacifies Obsessive Compulsive Disorder

Obsessive Compulsive Disorder or OCD drives a person to think repetitively about a certain incident or an object. Such thoughts constantly play across a person's mind and lead them to neglect their duties and their personal lives. The patient becomes anxious about a particular event and conducts a certain action over and over again. Their thoughts are occupied and their bodies refuse to break out of an obsessive reverie.

A very effective way to ease an OCD patient's anxiety, and to treat the inability to calm them down from a mind consuming thought is to use a spinner. This allows the patient to feel safe and secure without worrying about the numerous issues that may be present in their lives. The spinner provides a warm environment for the user by helping to relive stress and allow their mind to release the captivating thoughts.

## 9. Mimics a Massage

Using the spinner over the user's body distributes pressure evenly throughout their body. This has similar effects of a deep tissue massage. The pressure of the spinner goes deep within your tissues while you use it to fall asleep. A massage is supposed to help our body and mind relax – which can be easily done at home by using a weighted blanket. The physical factor of a massage might provide its own intimate yet soothing aspect, but the weighted blanket is proven to give you similar results to an actual massage in the long run.

## 10. Improves Cognitive Function

Taking a look at the overall therapeutic benefits of spinners, we can see that it relieves stress, reduces tension, induces sleep, calms your mind and relaxes your body. These components are very important if you want to live a healthy and happy life. Raised blood pressure, anxiety and lack of sleep are truly killers of productivity and normal behavior. Sleeping with the weighted blanket promotes the users overall well-being by ensuring that they tackle their daily issues with a clear head and a well-rested body. With a clear mind, a person's cognitive functions are improved. They are able to perform efficiently and effectively without being burdened by psychological issues and behavioral changes.

The highly astounding spinners promise the magical wonders of solving sleep issues, panic attacks, anxiety related disorders, lack of concentration and even aggressive behavioral problems that affect the smooth proceedings of one's daily life. You can enjoy the successful results of the spinners without the high costs of therapy sessions, drugs and sedatives that are traditionally used to pacify more tremulous patients. Give this effective and inexpensive spinner a try for one of the best night's sleep you've ever had in your life and feel great when you wake up every morning!

Fidget spinners are increasingly becoming popular as anxiety and stress-reduction tools every passing day. These low-cost, simple and effective toys have gained this immense popularity due to the internet, and are being used by millions of people worldwide now. For people suffering from ADD, autism, smoking, fidgeting, ADHD, nail biting, and other habits, they can be a good choice to get rid of those habits. They are also helpful as they offer an outlet for energy release and help in increasing calmness, focus and concentration levels.

The best part about hand fidget spinners is that these are compact, pocket-sized devices that can be carried around anywhere. Made from a variety of materials ranging from wood, metal and plastic, these come in a variety of shapes and sizes. There are also many different types available that are made with 3D printing technology. They have bearings made of wood or steel attached to them that makes them spin, making it an excellent stress reduction tool. I've reviewed some of the best hand fidget spinner toys on offer that you can go with.

## What are the different types of fidget spinners?

Different types of spinners are made up of different materials in their structures. Both the spinner and the bearings have their own material which has its own advantages and disadvantages. Depending on what each material has to offer, the price for the various fidget spinners also differ. The fidget spinners are made of numerous materials including steel, brass, copper, titanium, wood and they are even 3D printed. They have been divided as follows on the basis of their material:

**Superior quality:** These fidget spinners are made of steel, copper, titanium or brass come under this category. These are considered to be of high quality because of a lot of reasons. Firstly, they are super quiet which means you can play with them anywhere without annoying any people around you. Secondly, the weights on these are equally balanced which makes them rotate more smoothly and also for a longer period. These types of fidget spinners is the highest priced available in the market.

**Professional quality:** The models made out of wood come under this category because their wooden look gives a classy and professional perspective and hence make a nice addition to the office desk. Also, they are very lightweight and easy to carry. They last long just like the metal spinners. They tend to offer a great spinning time because they are lighter than the metal ones. They are more of a mid-priced fidget spinner.

**Cheap quality**: The models which are 3D printed come under this category because they are cheap and made out of a classic. They are least priced as compared to most of them available on the market. They aren't really durable and are prone to breaking. They are a little bit louder as compared to the others, but they are a great choice for trying them for the first time before buying the expensive ones.

A Fidget spinner iss till new to the market, so one should definitely try the most suited type at first to see if they work for them or not.

**Dual bar** – The dual bar is the simplest and most compact of all types. They are made of all materials including plastics. There are three bearings with the central one being used to hold the device.

**Tri-Bar** – The Tri-Bar has a few advantages over the dual bar. It owns the property of being flexible to the user which makes it more favorable. It is one of the most therapeutic devices which outsmart even dangerous and sometimes even costly medical practices.

**Quad-Bar** – The quad bar fidget spinner is the modified version of the tri-bar, with its extra bearings and flexibility.

This is used majorly by those patients with the highest levels of panic and anxiety.

**Custom Bar** – The custom and DIY types are reserved for those people who do not have the luxury to afford branded items. They are mainly made of any waste material by people who are not dedicated merely to the profession of producing these toys.

## What is the need for fidget spinners?

As mentioned above our world is slowly moving towards a style where one in a hundred of the people will have to admit themselves to a psychologist. The stress level experienced by the young people through their jobs, by parents while trying to mentor their rebellious teenagers, teens while trying to rebel through their lives and old people while trying to remain focused and energetic even if their body says no.

### Killing boredom

Often we find ourselves checking our phones a number of times during meetings, waiting for a date or even in the elevators. This can turn into an obsession at times. However, it can be solved if we are bright enough to keep a fidget spinner in our hands. This object gives us better focus and keeps our fingers busy thus preventing several of us from eating away our nails or getting up from our desks to visit the canteen a one hundred times in between office hours.

Some have also identified these objects to be an object of conversation. So, if you are waiting for a bus and spinning these toys in your hands, a pretty girl comes and asks you what you are doing! Well, thats one of the easiest ways to start off a budding friendship.

## Better focus and concentration

The finger fidgets are now being employed in hospitals and offices alike to improve the mental constitution of the patients as well as the employees. With the extremely attractive picture that it presents, it is next to impossible for a patient or a worker to ignore this object placed on his/her table. Patients suffering from concentration disorders and mild diseases like Autism, ADD or ADHD will find it increasingly easier to concentrate and understand all the things they are supposed to do. For workers who suffer from stress due to workload and other personal issues, this is one object where they can actually let out their frustration and built up negative energy in a productive manner.

## Overcoming addictions

The finger spinner help people who are trying to overcome their mild addictions like the annoying habit of desk drumming, nose cleansing, pencil tapping, nail biting, etc. Sometimes even smokers find it easier to get away from smoking by keeping their fingers occupied with these mini twirlers. The soothing effect often transfers the positive energy to the users thus pulling them away from their addictions.

## Tending overactive personalities

Some people often find it difficult to sit for hours in a place and often fidget and get restless. This is most common in the Autistic patients. They require the feeling of being in motion intermittently. These objects when in motion in their hands give them the feeling of a part of their body in motion, thus reducing their anxiety level and increasing their concentration on the subject in front of them.

## What to keep in mind while buying fidget spinners?

Nowadays, fidget spinners are available in the market from various manufacturers, all of them providing ones with varied advantages and uses. To select the one we actually require is the difficult task. This basic design features of this spinner are its speed, durability, compactness, cost, the material of bearing, rotation time, etc.

The essential details to keep in mind are –

**Actual need** – If the true necessity for the product is to increase the concentration of students or employees and to keep small children occupied, a smooth fidget spinner of no dual bar will do. As it is of low cost and of high effectiveness in a small range, this object is the perfect solution to it. But if we are looking to treat a serious illness like autism or ADD or a smoking disorder, then a high speed, high quality and highly durable fidget spinner will be necessary.

**Basic materials** – The material of its cover and bearing plays a significant role in the durability. For example, the highly Ceramic Silicon Nitride used in the bearings of smooth fidget spinner which betters steel bearings, the lightweight aluminum material employed in certain types which are more durable, the ABS plastic frame spinner which is ultra durable, the EDC 7D custom models with their dirt repellents are unique in their own ways. The different materials used for manufacturing like copper, brass, etc. have to be taken into account while concluding on their effectiveness.

**Bearings** – The best one in the market are considered to be the ABEC -11 type bearings. They are used in EDC customs dirt repellant spinners. These have to resist the spinning moment and also offer less friction to trapped dirt.
So, the hand spinner is basically made up of different shapes, sizes and cost. Regardless of all this, they are most useful for all people from different areas of life. Infant these toys are even kept in the showcases since they resemble the UFO which makes the kids even more curious about them.

# Raptor R1 Fidget Spinner Tri-Spinner Fidget Toy

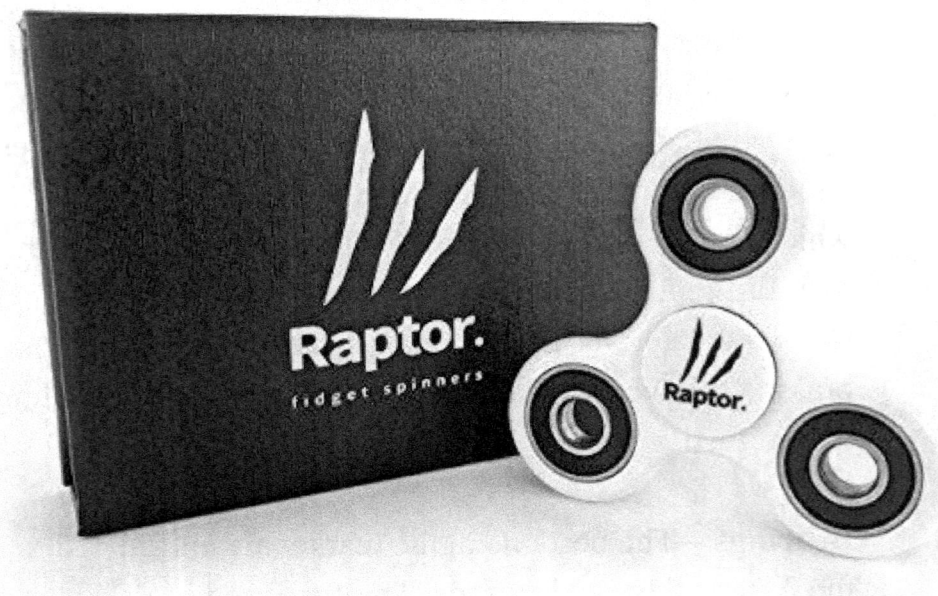

Too occupied with the stress on your mind? Or is it the anxiety that has been keeping you from focusing on your work? Well, you don't have to worry about these petty distractions anymore. The new Raptor R1 fidget spinner is here to make things easier in your life. The triune fidget spinner comes with high-speed tri fidget spinner technology which is the talk of the town. This fidget is a toy stress reducer that comes along with premium bearing. This is a

Therapeutic Benefits of Fidget Spinners!

perfect product for ADHD, ADD, Autism Adult Children as well as Anxiety.

The hand spinner is specially designed in such a way that it can comfortably adapt to any sorts of fingers that users can probably have. The device comes with excellent ceramic bearings built in it for having a better grip on the product. This is a high-quality fidget spinner toy stresser guarantees that the caps and bearings will not be severe from the product unless it is you only who decides to get them out. The spinner has a sleek frame which is unbreakable as well as injection molded. There are no 3D prints on the spinner to keep the super smooth ceramic surface of the bearing friction free for maintaining its quality.

This is an amazingly fast spinner fidget that will surely satisfy the restlessness growing within you. The spinner is really smooth and fast as it has been noticed that it can spin on an average for about 3 minutes continuously, but then again this duration will vary from person to person as it depends upon the power that one applies to rotate it.

The product by Raptor Fidget Spinners is only sold by Raptor and all the products or items that are shipped, the FBA ships them. Further, there is a guarantee of 2-day delivery which is pretty cool because it is really hard to stay away from something so cool after youve ordered it.

# Zekpro The Anti-Anxiety 360 Spinner Helps Focusing Fidget Toys

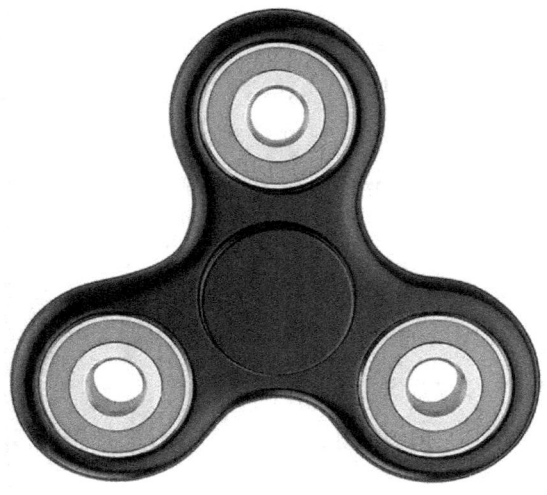

We all have that habit of keep doing something or the other with our fingers even when we are already busy doing some work (be it merely thinking only). To deal with this habit of keeping your fingers up to something, this spinner toy fidget is a must thing that every individual should think of gifting themselves.

Once you conquer anxiety, consider that you have already found the solution to half of the problems that you have. Hence, this toy! Even though it falls to be in the category of a toy, do not take this Zekpro anti-anxiety 360 spinner lightly. The fidget hand spinner helps an individual in bringing out the best in him simply by letting him deal with issues such as stress, anxiety or be it the depressing thoughts that seem to cloud your mind and vision. All these issues greatly hinder individuals performance, but with this premium quality EDC Focus toy, it can all be dealt with easily. The 3D fidget is a high-quality product that can be used by both kids as well as adults to fight their anxiety problem. Not that it is merely a stress buster, but also it is an excellent play thing to pass your time with. Deep thinkers or people who like to indulge in creativity can find this fidget spinner tool to be really useful in awakening their brighter side.

This super is easily portable fidget promises to be there in your pocket even when you do not have pennies in there because of its highly mobile nature. In addition to that, this stress-reducing device comes with a really smooth surface that it makes it really easy for users to handle and use. The rounded edges of the fidget spinner are smooth and comfortable while spinning. The one plus point that this quick spinner offers is the Premium Si3n4 ceramic bearings that is a high-speed bearing that promises user a firm grip over the spinner which in turn enhances their experience while using it. The average duration for which such a spinner could spin has been noted to be 1 to 3 minutes.

# Hysada Spinner Fidget Toy, Fidget Spinner Focus Toy for Autism

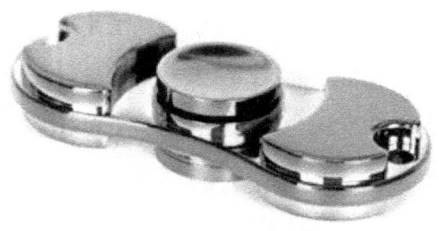

It is very common for a person to go through stress and anxiety in his day to day life. Being occupied by a hectic and tiring schedule every day, people learn living with stress instead of tackling it, and this causes their lives to become boring and dull. Hysada has launched HysadaSpinnerFidget toy, which is a fidget spinner focus toy which is made of aluminium and offers high speed spins to tackle your anxiety or stress. It is a fantastic hand spinner to fight stress, increase your focus, to quit bad habits, having deep thoughts or working with a creative mind.

Being made of aluminum, the Hysada Spinner fidget is a very light and durable and has a very comfortable feel to suit your hands. Its smooth surface finish makes it very easy to handle and used to relieve your anxiety without hurting your hands. It doesn't even require any maintenance. No repair oil, no water, no alcohol or anything is needed to clean it. It works straight out of the box. Here's a tip, if you feel like the toy is loose, then just remove the stainless cap, tighten it and put it back on and you're good to go. Also, the toy is very easy to carry and easy to use. It has no noise generation to keep your mind calm. Because of the light weight material used to design it, the toy would make your stress and anxiety go away without disturbing the people around you.

The Hysada Spinner fidget is very easy to use. You just need to simply hold the spinner with one hand and the other hand to give it continuous small strikes to keep the spinning going on indefinitely. You will need some practice to keep the action going, but once you get the hold of it, it becomes so easy and relaxing. It doesn't take much time to be a skillful spinner. You'll find yourself spinning it for hours, and it will help your stress go away without even you getting any idea.

# AMILIFE EDC Fidget Spinner High Speed Stainless Steel Bearing

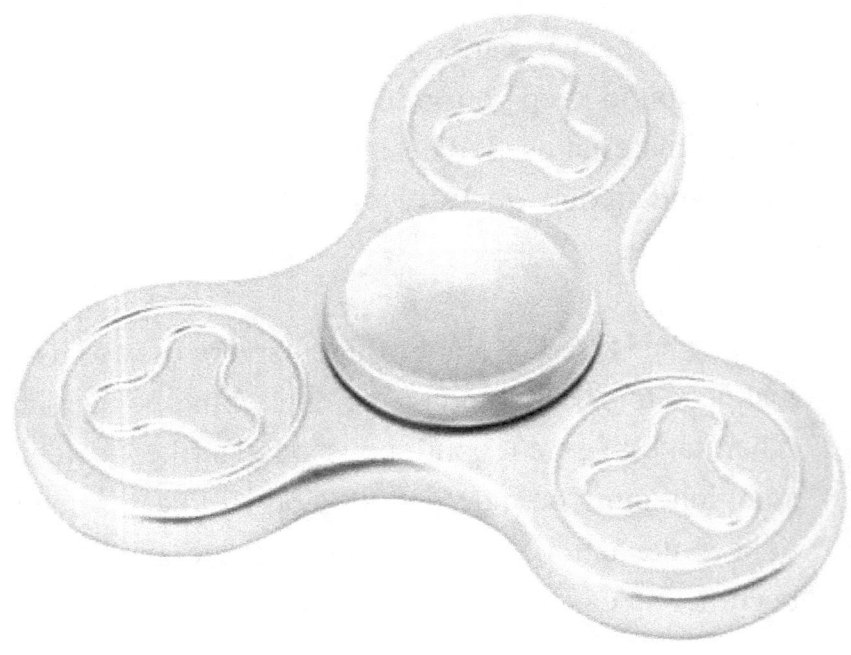

You have been up all night trying to find some sleep or if not that, then something to do. These hard insomniac times have always made things only harder and more difficult for us individuals. Well, the solution to these problems is right here the AMILIFE EDC Fidget Spinner High-Speed Stainless Steel Bearings.

The AMILIFE EDC fidget Spinner comes in flashy golden color with very catchy looks. It is of the size of 7 cm with a thickness of about 1 cm. This is a heavy weighing spinner, and its heavy weight is a plus point as it enhances the speed of the spinner. Also, it helps the spinner in keep spinning for a longer duration. The user can hold the spinner in one hand and rotate with the other. Although, experienced fidget spinner users may not need the help of another hand and comfortable turn it using one hand only.

The EDC Fidget can rotation an average for about a period of one to three minutes which is great. This will help the ADD, and ADHD sufferers and not just that, people who are facing anxiety, sleep-depravity, etc. can all be benefitted from this anxiety relief toy. Also, it helps in aiming at your goals and having a prolonged focus. The center of the fastest fidget spinner has ceramic center bearings with SLA technology for a better experience of the users.

# Holisouse Tri-Spinner Fidget Hand Spinner Toy Stress Reducer EDC

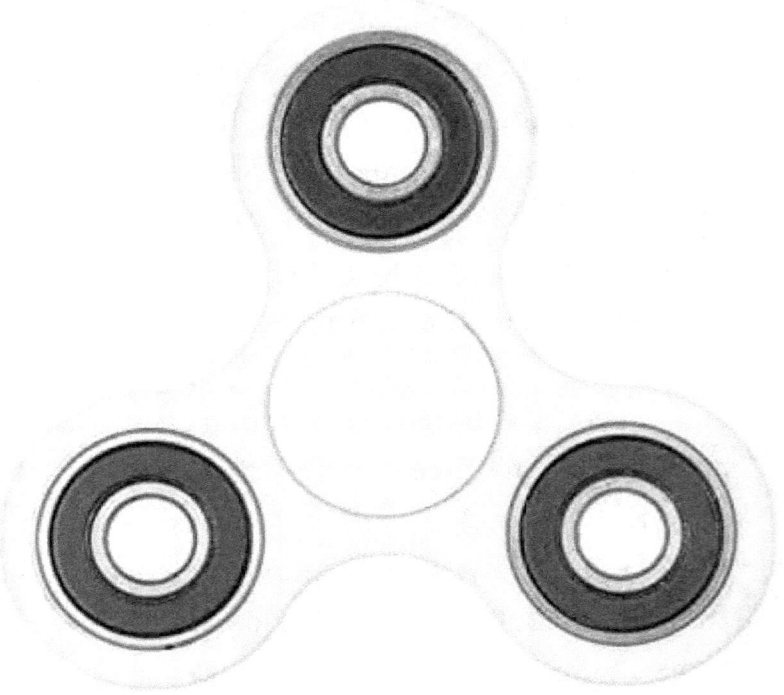

The Holisouse Tri-Spinner Fidget Hand Spinner Toy is injection molded from ABS plastic which is a stronger and environmentally friendly material that also gives longer service. It has a fantastic finish and a very high shatter resistance in comparison to other 3D spinners. The ZrO2

---

hybrid ceramic bearings in the center allows it to perform better and helps rotate effortlessly in our hands for at least 3 minutes. The three additional bearings on the sides have been chosen due to their increased weight which provides the spinner with extra inertia and spinning momentum that helps in longer spins. Each bearing also provides greater fidgeting fun.

The Spinner comfortably fits in your pocket and is easy to carry around. It also helps provoke deeper thoughts and increase concentration and focus. It is light and highly durable. For kids and adults with sensitive hands, its smooth edges prove to be handy. The spinner is non-irritant and improves mental focus in people having ADD or ADHD. The spinner also does not make any sound and is quiet. It has a very sturdy construction, and the buttons feel good. The spinner spins without any efforts with a smooth movement. The bearings are removable and easy to clean. This spinner outperforms the expensive ones in the market.

The Tri-Spinner helps you stop distracting people by fidgeting. It does not require any oiling or maintenance. The design is simple, but one spin will keep you hooked. The motion is also nearly frictionless. The spinner is very easy to use. However, it takes a little time to get adjusted to it.

# Toplay Fidget Spinner Toy Stress Reducer Ceramic Bearing

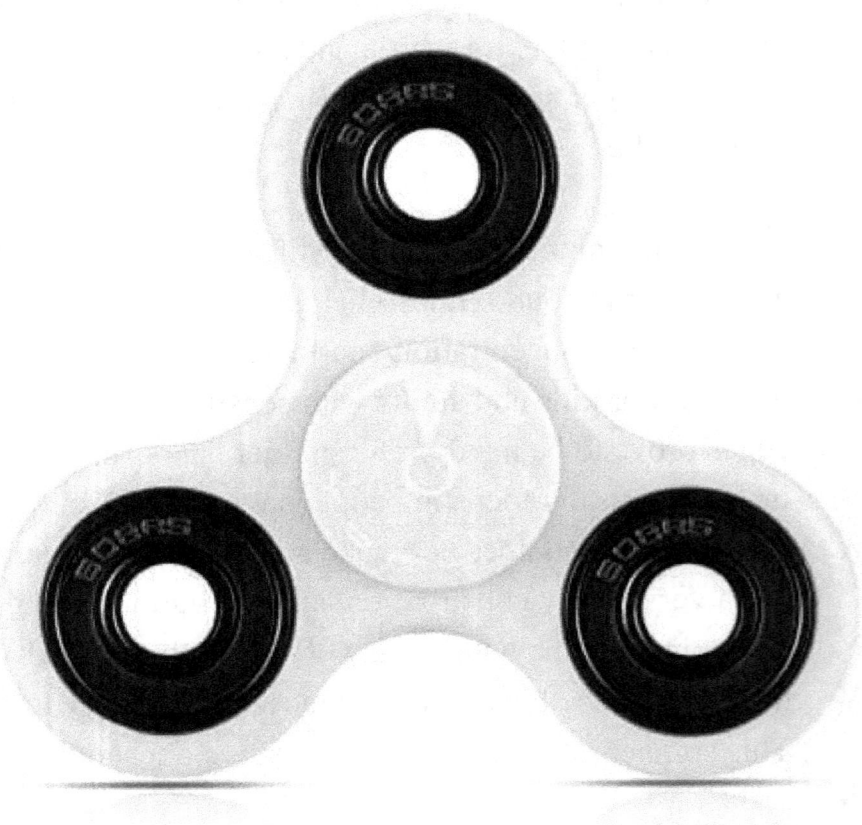

The Toplay Spinner Stress Reducer is perfect for ADHD, ADD, stress, anxiety and adult autism. One should definitely prefer this toy to tackle his obstacles that hinder his growth. It has been suggested by a lot of users that the effectiveness of the ToplayFidget Spinner is unbeatable.

It is made of ultra-durable ABS plastic body and is non 3-d printed. The latest low friction technology has been used to make the bearings by incorporating ceramic bearing to ensure longevity and smooth rotation. This spinner is easy to carry, small, discrete and fun. It also guarantees to rotate for more than 1+ minute. Also, the it's available in a wide range of colors for you to choose from as per your likes.

If you wish to quit bad habits or you want help with your anxiety, Fidgets, focusing, ADHD, Autism or staying awake, the ToplayFidgetSpinner Stress Reducer is a great toy for you. Like every other spinning Fidget toys, the ToplayFidgetspinner also takes spinning or breaking in to achieve higher spinning times. It lasts according to the duration you take to turn it. So, the more you spin, it will last more time. It has a professional inline skate 608 bearings and ceramic balls which are premium and hence the ball is able to give a 1+ minute spinning time. Also, if you clean the bearings of the toy, it will last longer in spinning.

To rotate the ToplayFidgetSpinner toy stress reducer ceramic bearing, one must refer to the right way to achieve longer rotation times. To have longer spinning times, hold it in one hand and spin it continuously and rapidly using small constant strikes using the other hand to keep it spinning for long periods of time. Fingers of only one hand can be used to stop or resume spinning.

# NEW 7D Customs EDC Spinner Tri- Fidget Toy

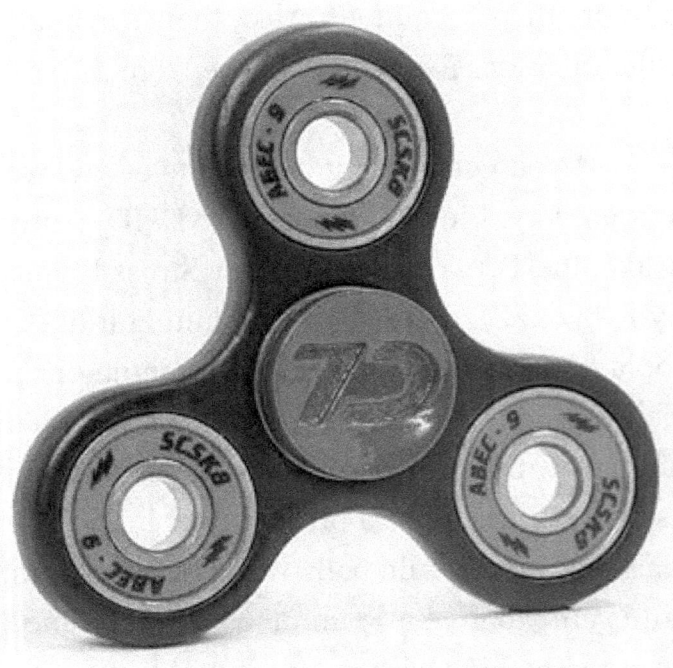

Do you click your pen when you are anxious? Do you tap your feet or hands on the table? Is your body on vibrate mode when you start to lose focus? If you answered yes to the above questions, then the 7D Customs EDC Spinner Tri-Fidget toy is the one for you. A fidget toy helps to increase your focus by centering your energy with the spinning motion of the toy. So, by concentrating on the movement of the toy, you can reduce your habits of fidgeting. For all those out there who have ADD or ADHD or even just looking to break a bad habit, this toy is the right fit for you.

The 7D Customs EDC Spinner 2017 model is rated as one of the best fidget spinner toys in the market for producing the longest spins with a higher durability rate. This model comes in two colours. The body is completely black or white depending on your choice of colour, and the outer ball bearing is orange with black accents. The body of the toy is made of high-quality plastic and not 3-D printed like some of the cheaper ones. The dealer ensures that each toy is handmade with utmost care and they have all undergone precision testing in the U.S before they are shipped to the buyer. The outer bearings are sealed, and the one in the middle is made with a top grade Abec 9 bearings with a finger grip that offers better handling and increases the ease of use.

Another notable feature of the 7D Customs model is that it has a dirt resistant finish that offers protection against dust, grime, and scratch marks. Since the product is meant to be handled with our hands, it is easy to get dust on it and even score up the finish, but not on this model. It is easy to clean the toy, and the sheen lasts longer than most of the plastic toys in the market.

The product also has a nice feel as the overall weight of the product comes to 131 g (0.29 lb), and the weight is distributed evenly. The performance of the Abec 9 bearings leads to a faster, smoother, and a longer lasting spin. The spin rate of the toy averages from 60 to 90 seconds with little to no noise and with a steady spin. Overall, the product delivers on the promise of a nearly indestructible spinner toy for those fidgeting hands.

# VICTOREM EDC Hand Spinner Metal Fidget ADHD Focus Toy

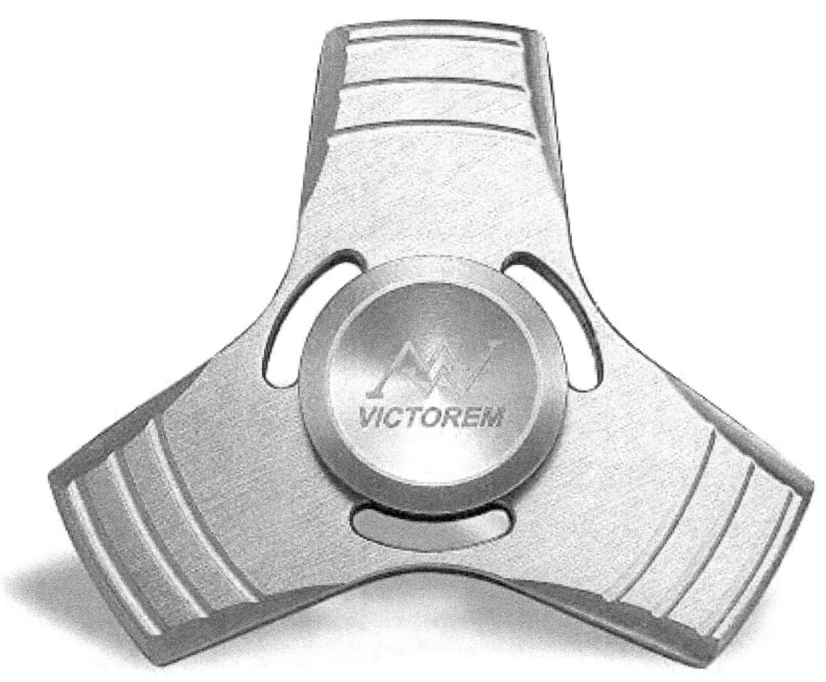

For all those wishing to increase their focus and hoping to overcome the urge to bite their nails, or twirl their hair look no further as the VICTOREM EDC Hand Spinner Metal fidget is the one you are looking for. The spinner helps to provide an instant comfort and over a period will replace the unwanted motion or movement that is linked to the urge that one is trying to break. The VICTOREM EDC metal fidget spinner is different from most of the available ones in the fact that it is made entirely of metal and thus provides a longer spinning and a more sturdy design.

The body of the fidget toy is made of copper and brass, and this gives the spinner the added strength and stability to go on for longer spinning times. It is sturdy, so there are no problems of breakage. The body has a lovely rose gold tone with the center grip in a metallic gold tone. The bearings inside the middle grip are made of ceramic and are cage-less, so they tend to produce a slight noise as they spin. The spinner weighs around 75 g(0.16 lb) and the overall weight distribution on the spinner is equal. The size is compact, and it fits snugly in your hand and can be handled with one hand given enough practice. The edges are not sharp, so there are no chances of any accidental injury.

The spinning time out of the box averages to 5 minutes but can last longer still. If the spin-rate declines, it can be adjusted by tightening the metal piece inside the cap. This part loosens the longer the product is used, so by tightening it, you can extend the spinning duration of the toy for far longer than 5 minutes. All the parts are removable and can be easily assembled back. Since the spinner bearings are cage-less, it is best not to be handled by children below the age of 8 as it can cause a choking hazard. In comparison with its plastic-made counterparts, it offers a better durability to the toy. Its size lends it some innocuousness that allows you to play withit in any sort of location such as a work environment or even during class lectures without any disturbance.

## <u>Vafru Fidget Cube,Vafru Mini Magic Cube</u>

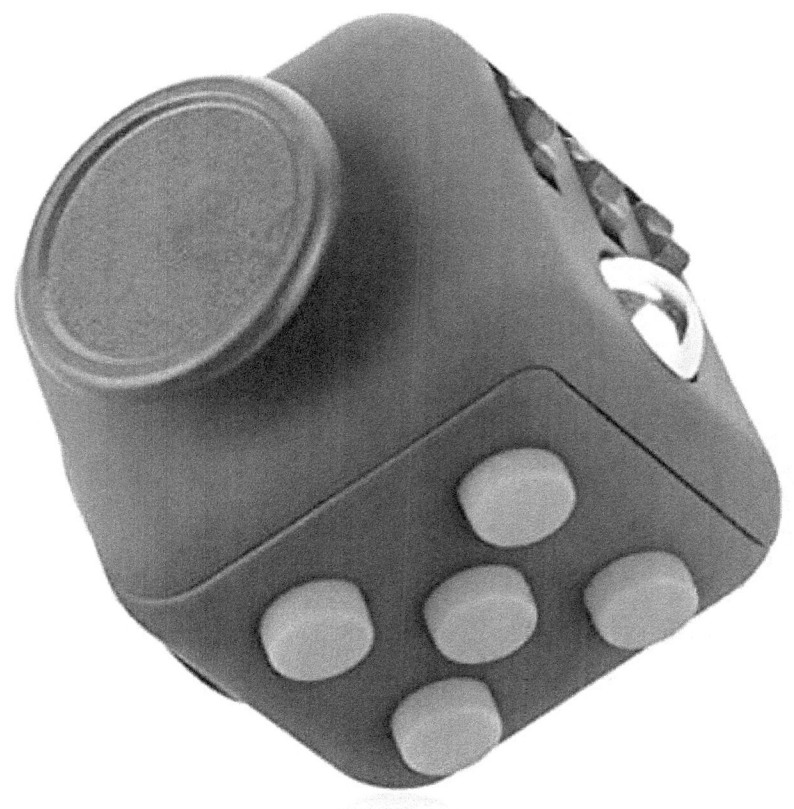

With great power comes great responsibility and with that comes greater anxiety. We are surrounded by many stress-inducing factors at school, work, or even at home. Children are finding it harder to focus without the need to fidget about in place. So, to solve this problem of hyper anxiety Vafru has introduced a new decompression toy: the Fidget Cube, a pocket fidget toy. The Vafru Mini Magic Anti-anxiety dice cube is a one of a kind toy that provides six different ways to help channel your excess energy in a more constructive and less obtrusive way.

The Mini Magic cube is made of high-grade plastic and measures 3.3 x 3.3 x 3.3 cm (1.29 x 1.29 x 1.29 in) in size. Each face of the cube offers a diverse method of stress-relief. One side there is a small joystick that allows a similar gliding motion that can soothe all the game lovers and gamer enthusiasts alike. Another side has a series of five buttons arranged in the form of an x and can be clicked. Three of them provide a clicking sound to soothe the clicker in all of us while the other two are silenced. There is also a round dial for those that want to move their thumb in a soothing, circular motion. A giant switch on one side of the cube can be turned on and off in slow motion for a silent click or faster for a more audible sound effect. One face of the cube has three gears and a ball that can also be clicked. The bottom of the cube has a groove that can be rubbed. This works on the principle of the worry stones that can help relieve anxiety when it is rubbed.

The Magic Cube comes is a wide variety of colors, but the theme is a black body with the buttons and other elements in differing color schemes. It is also available at an affordable price and is a beneficial addition to anyone's desk. The cube is tiny and can be handled with ease.

www.ingramcontent.com/pod-product-compliance
Lightning Source LLC
Chambersburg PA
CBHW072019290526
45787CB00013B/1343